Kreative Juicing:

A Natural Guide to Wellness

Kreative Juicing:

A Natural Guide to Wellness

BALOWZOOM
BOOKS

Zakiya Grier

An Original Publication of BALOWZOOM BOOKS

Identifiers: ISBN 979-8-9923204-5-9 (Paperback)
ISBN 979-8-9923204-4-2 (E-book)
Balow zoom website.

Cover Art by LaVar J. Henry Jr.
Visit bzoombooks.com for contact information
@Kreatively.Kiy Instagram
@KreativelyKiy TikTok
@KreativelyKiy Facebook

Dedication

Hi Mommy,
This is Zakiya and I love you so much!

Introduction

Kreatively Kiy is a versatile and dynamic business offering a wide range of services. Here is where creativity meets wellness in every form! From sweet treats to personalized gifts that don't miss a beat, Kreatively Kiy is built on the belief that creativity can transform lives- inside and out. Our mission is rooted in bringing happiness to those we encounter. This juicing guide is a direct offset of this vision, exercising the fact that we must nourish our body and surroundings with equal importance. If you look good, then you will feel good, which will lead you to do good in whatever you may face. Through healthy vibrant juices, you're challenged to experience wellness from the inside out! People often state "You are what you eat". Let's eat great so we can be great! A Kreatively inspired life must begin with a grounded, healthy foundation.

Table of Contents

How to Use This Book

Brought to you with love by Kreatively Kiy LLC

Welcome to your wellness journey one vibrant, nourishing sip at a time!

This book was crafted with intention by Kreatively Kiy, a brand that lives at the intersection of creativity and wellness. From handcrafted treats to personalized art and lifestyle design, our mission will always be to uplift and inspire inside and out. This juicing guide is a natural extension of that mission: to help you look good, feel good, and do good, starting from within.

Whether you're new to juicing or looking to spice up your routine, this book is here to empower, educate, and energize you. Each recipe is thoughtfully created with ingredients that fuel the body, support long-term health, and taste absolutely amazing.

About the Juice Yields

All recipes in this book have been tested using a **GDOR 1200W Centrifugal Juicer**, yielding an average of **70—80 ounces** per batch. Please note that different juicers can produce different yields. **Cold-press juicers** tend to extract more liquid, especially from leafy greens, while **blenders with straining** can vary based on technique.

Think of our yields as flexible guides not rules. Use what you have, do what you can, and adjust as needed.

Tips for Getting the Most Out of This Book:

- **Start slow.** Try one juice every few days, then build consistency.

- **Prep ahead.** Wash, cut, and portion your produce in advance for easy juicing.
- **Make it yours.** Don't be afraid to swap ingredients based on what your body needs or what's in season.
- **Listen to your body.** Wellness isn't one -size-fits-all it's about finding what makes *you* feel your best.
- **Drink with intention.** Use this time to check in with yourself, your energy, and your goals.

Our Hope for You

At Kreatively Kiy, we believe that wellness is the foundation for everything you create in your body, your home, and your life. We hope this book not only adds color to your fridge, but also joy to your heart and fuel to your purpose.

Now grab your favorite glass, get your juicer ready, and let's pour into the best version of you.

SECTION I

Energizing Morning Juices

FreshFuel Fusion

Ingredients

- 2 cups of water
- 2 whole pineapples
- 16oz of strawberries
- 2 whole mangoes
- 1 head of celery
- 9oz spinach
- 2 cucumbers
- 2 lemons
- 5 green apples
- ½ lb green grapes

Instructions

1. Wash all produce thoroughly.
2. Peel or core ingredients as needed (e.g., pineapples, mangoes, apples).
3. Cut larger fruits or vegetables into smaller chunks for easier juicing.
4. Juice all ingredients using a juicer of your choice (then strain).
5. Stir well, chill if desired, and enjoy fresh!

Pro Tip: Chill your produce beforehand or add ice after juicing for a cooler, more refreshing drink.

Yield

Approximately 76 ounces (about 9—10 servings)

Storage

- Store in an airtight glass container in the refrigerator.
- Best consumed within **24 to 72 hours** for peak freshness and nutritional value.

Kreatively Kiy's Notes

This juice is perfect for providing early morning energy boosts!

Root&Rind

Ingredients

- 3 cups of watermelon, cubed
- 1 whole beet
- 5 red crisp apples
- 2 lemons
- 16oz of medjool dates
- 1 cup of coconut water
- 3 (3-inch) pieces fresh ginger
- 4—5 sprigs fresh mint

Instructions

1. Wash all produce thoroughly.
2. Peel or core ingredients as needed (e.g., beets, lemons, apples).
3. Cut larger fruits or vegetables into smaller chunks for easier juicing.
4. Juice all ingredients using a juicer of your choice (then strain).
5. Stir well, chill if desired, and enjoy fresh!

Pro Tip: Mint is **powerful**, but it's also **refreshing** and balances strong flavors like ginger and lemon. You can adjust up or down easily without altering the recipe too much.

Yield

Approximately 102 ounces (about 10—11 servings)

Storage

- Store in an airtight glass container in the refrigerator.
- Best consumed within **24 to 72 hours** for peak freshness and nutritional value.

Kreatively Kiy's Notes

Rise and shine with Root&Rind! Drink this earthy yet refreshing juice in the morning to boost heart health, energy, and support gut health.

pHresh Formula

Ingredients

- 1 bunch of kale
- 1 bunch of radish tops
- 5 cucumbers
- 5 green apples
- 2 (3-inch) pieces fresh ginger
- 5 bartlett pears
- Honey (optional)
- 1 cups of water
- 3 lemons

Instructions

1. Wash all produce thoroughly.
2. Peel or core ingredients as needed (e.g., lemons, apples).
3. Cut larger fruits or vegetables into smaller chunks for easier juicing.
4. Juice all ingredients using a juicer of your choice (then strain).
5. Stir well, chill if desired, and enjoy fresh!

Pro Tip: Ginger juice is **POTENT** strong and spicy. Start small if you're unsure.

Yield

Approximately 50 ounces (about 5-6 servings)

Storage

- Store in an airtight glass container in the refrigerator.
- Best consumed within **24 to 72 hours** for peak freshness and nutritional value.

Kreatively Kiy's Notes

Feel a wave of freshness jolt through your body as you indulge in this energy drink without the caffeine! This juice supports immunity and pH balance all while leaving your skin glowing.

Citrus Reign

Ingredients

- 5 guavas
- 3 starfruit
- 1 head of celery
- 2 (3-inch) pieces fresh ginger (optional)
- 4oz bag of watercress
- 4 oranges

Instructions

1. Wash all produce thoroughly.
2. Peel or core ingredients as needed (e.g., guava, oranges, remove celery ends).
3. Cut larger fruits or vegetables into smaller chunks for easier juicing.
4. Juice all ingredients using a juicer of your choice (then strain).
5. Stir well, chill if desired, and enjoy fresh!

Pro Tip: Add a sprig of mint or a splash of lime to enhance the citrusy brightness and mellow the ginger's warmth.

Yield

Approximately 88—92 ounces (about 9—10 servings)

Storage

- Store in an airtight glass container in the refrigerator.
- Best consumed within **24 to 72 hours** for peak freshness and nutritional value.

Kreatively Kiy's Notes

Claim your crown Citrus Reign rules the realm of energy, flavor, and flawless mornings

BALOWZOOM
BOOKS

The 8th and 13th pages in physical books are intentionally left blank as a nuanced homage to my roots in Tampa, represented by the 813-area code. This empty page symbolizes the power of presence and silence.

The spaces where creativity, reflection, and meaning are born. Just as my city shaped me, these pauses in the book allow readers to shape their own thoughts and interpretations, making the journey uniquely personal. It's our quiet signature, a tribute, and an invitation all at once.

Golden Bloom

Ingredients

- 2 (3-inch) pieces fresh turmeric
- 1 papaya
- 1 head of bok choy
- 5 passion fruit
- 1 Soursop
- 1 Pineapple

Pro Tip: A squeeze of lime can lift the tropical flavor and add extra freshness!

Yield

Approximately 90—95 ounces (about 9—10 servings)

Instructions

1. Wash all produce thoroughly.
2. Peel or core ingredients as needed (e.g., pineapples, papaya, separate leaves and stems).
3. Juicing passion fruit:
   a. Slice each passion fruit in half.
   b. Scoop the pulp and seeds into a fine mesh strainer over a bowl.
   c. Press with a spoon to release the juice; discard the seeds
4. Juice all ingredients using a juicer of your choice (then strain).
5. Add passion fruit juice and soursop pieces to juice.
6. Stir well, chill if desired, and enjoy fresh!

Storage

- Store in an airtight glass container in the refrigerator.
- Best consumed within **24 to 72 hours** for peak freshness and nutritional value.

Kreatively Kiy's Notes

Golden Bloom shines with vibrant tropical energy. Soursop adds a creamy texture that makes this juice feel indulgent yet light. Drink in the morning or mid-day to support digestion, circulation, and sustained natural energy all day long.

SECTION II

Detox and Cleanse Juices

Pearberry Pop

Ingredients

- 32oz organic cranberry juice
- 5 fresh okra pods, thinly sliced (for infusion)
- 4 lemons
- 2 cups of water
- Agave
- 5 red crisp apples
- 5 red Anjou pears
- 1 whole pineapple

Instructions

1. Wash all produce thoroughly.
2. Peel or core ingredients as needed (e.g., pineapples, lemons, apples).
3. Cut larger fruits or vegetables into smaller chunks for easier juicing.
4. Juice all ingredients (excluding okra) using a juicer of your choice (then strain).
5. Stir sliced okra into the juice
6. Stir well, chill if desired, and enjoy fresh!

Pro Tip: For a stronger **mucilaginous (gel-like)** effect, let the okra sit in the juice longer up to 30 minutes in the fridge.

Serving Size

Approximately 80 ounces (about 8-9 servings)

Storage

- Store in an airtight glass container in the refrigerator.
- Best consumed within **24 to 72 hours** for peak freshness and nutritional value.

Kreatively Kiy's Notes

Let's pop into the fact that this juice is a power house fuel for the body! A drink that supports digestive health, kidney health, heart health, and immunity all in one!

Berry Bold

Ingredients

- 3 red grapefruits
- 2 cups of raspberries
- 2 cups of blackberries
- 1 small watermelon
- 1 beet
- Agave (optional)

Instructions

1. Wash all produce thoroughly.
2. Peel or core ingredients as needed (e.g., grapefruit, beets, watermelon).
3. Cut larger fruits or vegetables into smaller chunks for easier juicing.
4. Juice all ingredients using a juicer of your choice (then strain).
5. Stir in desired amount of agave nectar until fully dissolved.
6. Stir well, chill if desired, and enjoy fresh!

Pro Tip: For a bolder flavor, let the juice rest for 10—15 minutes before chilling—the beet's earthiness and berry sweetness will deepen beautifully.

Serving Size

Approximately **85 ounces** (about 8—9 servings)

Storage

- Store in an airtight glass container in the refrigerator.
- Best consumed within **24 to 72 hours** for peak freshness and nutritional value.

Kreatively Kiy's Notes

Drink Berry Bold and watch your energy, mood, and mirror all say — "Oh, we did that."

Dragonberry Delight

Ingredients

- 2 red flesh dragonfruit
- 1 cup lychees, peeled and pitted
- 2 cups strawberries
- 3 kiwis

Instructions

1. Wash all produce thoroughly.
2. Peel or core ingredients as needed (e.g., kiwi, dragonfruit, lychee).
3. Cut larger fruits or vegetables into smaller chunks for easier juicing.
4. Juice all ingredients using a juicer of your choice (then strain).
5. Stir well, chill if desired, and enjoy fresh!

Pro Tip: For a slightly tropical twist, blend briefly with ice before serving.

Serving Size

Approximately 75 ounces (about 7—8 servings)

Storage

- Store in an airtight glass container in the refrigerator.
- Best consumed within **24 to 72 hours** for peak freshness and nutritional value.

Kreatively Kiy's Notes

Let Dragonberry Delight remind you that cleansing can taste deliciously magical.

Papaya Pineapple Twist

Ingredients

- 5 limes
- 1 papaya
- 1 pineapple
- 3 sprigs of mint leaves
- 2 large carrots
- 3 oranges

Instructions

1. Wash all produce thoroughly.
2. Peel or core ingredients as needed (e.g., pineapples, limes, papaya, oranges).
3. Cut larger fruits or vegetables into smaller chunks for easier juicing.
4. Juice all ingredients using a juicer of your choice (then strain).
5. Stir well, chill if desired, and enjoy fresh!

Pro Tip: Freeze leftover juice in ice cube trays perfect for quick smoothies or refreshing drinks.

Serving Size

Approximately 48—56 ounces (about 4—5 servings)

Storage

- Store in an airtight glass container in the refrigerator.
- Best consumed within **24 to 72 hours** for peak freshness and nutritional value.

Kreatively Kiy's Notes

This juice is basically a tropical vacation in a glass, giving your digestion, immunity, and taste buds a first-class upgrade all while detoxing and cleansing your body!

Berry Glow Cleanse

Ingredients

- 3 limes
- 2 cups of blueberries
- 1 pomegranate
- 1 cup organic prune juice
- 2 cucumbers
- 4 honey crisp apples

Instructions

1. Wash all produce thoroughly.
2. Peel or core ingredients as needed (e.g., limes, pomegranates, apples).
3. Cut larger fruits or vegetables into smaller chunks for easier juicing.
4. Juice all ingredients using a juicer of your choice (then strain).
5. Stir well, chill if desired, and enjoy fresh!

Pro Tip: For a gentle natural detox, let the juice sit for 10—15 minutes to allow the flavors and cleansing properties to meld.

Serving Size

Approximately 85 ounces (about 8—9 servings)

Storage

- Store in an airtight glass container in the refrigerator.
- Best consumed within **24 to 72 hours** for peak freshness and nutritional value.

Kreatively Kiy's Notes

Berry Glow Cleanse is your delicious daily reset hydrating, detoxifying, and turning every sip into a power move for your body.

SECTION III

Hydration and Beauty Juices

Waistline Wakeup

Ingredients

- 3 carrots
- 3 mangoes
- 3 oranges
- 1 (4-inch) piece fresh turmeric
- 1 (3-inch) piece fresh ginger
- 2 lemons
- Cayenne pepper (optional)
- 2 cucumber
- 3 honey crisp apples
- 2 cups of water

Instructions

1. Wash all produce thoroughly.
2. Peel or core ingredients as needed (e.g., oranges, mangoes, apples, lemons).
3. Cut larger fruits or vegetables into smaller chunks for easier juicing.
4. Juice all ingredients using a juicer of your choice (then strain).
5. Stir well, chill if desired, and enjoy fresh!

Pro Tip: For a smoother juicing process and better flavor balance, let the mangoes and oranges sit at room temperature for 10—15 minutes before juicing to release more juice and natural sweetness.

Yield

Approximately 70 ounces (about 7 servings)

Storage

- Store in an airtight glass container in the refrigerator.
- Best consumed within **24 to 72 hours** for peak freshness and nutritional value.

Kreatively Kiy's Notes

Spice things up with a pinch of cayenne and fresh ginger this fiery duo wakes you up, slims you down, and adds a glow that coffee never could.

Citrus Goldrush

Ingredients

- 3 oranges
- 2 ruby red grapefruit
- 2 lemons
- 4 limes
- 5 tangerines
- 1 pineapple
- Honey or agave
- 4—5 sprigs fresh mint
- 1 stalk lemongrass, bruised and chopped

Instructions

1. Wash all produce thoroughly.
2. Peel or core ingredients as needed (e.g., pineapples, lemons, oranges, grapefruits, limes).
3. Cut larger fruits or vegetables into smaller chunks for easier juicing.
4. Juice all ingredients using a juicer of your choice (then strain).
5. Stir well, chill if desired, and enjoy fresh!

Pro Tip: Roll your citrus fruits firmly on the countertop before juicing to unlock extra juice and boost flavor without any extra effort!

Yield

Makes approximately 80 ounces (7-8 servings)

Storage

- Store in an airtight glass container in the refrigerator.
- Best consumed within **24 to 72 hours** for peak freshness and nutritional value.

Kreatively Kiy's Notes

Catch the Goldrush for glowing skin Vitamin C fuels collagen production to keep your skin firm, smooth, and luminous.

Green Peace

Ingredients

- 10 ounces of spinach
- 5 green apples
- 2 cucumbers
- 2 lemons
- 1 pineapple
- Half an aloe vera leaf
- 1lb green grapes
- 1 cup of coconut water
- 5 fresh cinnamon sticks (for infusion)

Instructions

1. Wash all produce thoroughly.
2. Peel or core ingredients as needed (e.g., pineapples, mangoes, apples).
3. Cut larger fruits or vegetables into smaller chunks for easier juicing.
4. Juice all ingredients using a juicer of your choice (then strain).
5. Add cinnamon sticks to the freshly prepared juice, let it steep for 10—15 minutes (or longer for a stronger flavor) in the refrigerator, then remove before serving.
6. Stir well, chill if desired, and enjoy fresh!

Pro Tip: Let cinnamon sticks gently steep in your juice to add a warm, cozy touch that makes every sip feel refreshing and special.

Yield

Makes approximately 80 ounces (7-8 servings)

Storage

- Store in an airtight glass container in the refrigerator.
- Best consumed within **24 to 72 hours** for peak freshness and nutritional value.

Kreatively Kiy's Notes

The cinnamon stick infusion is used to elevate your juice with a subtle warmth that refreshes while gently supporting digestion.

Tropical Glow Lemonade

Ingredients

- 2 cups fresh sugarcane juice (see sub-recipe below)
- 10 lemons
- 6 oranges
- 2 cups of water
- 2 sprigs of mint leaves

Instructions

1. Peel the sugarcane using a sharp knife or vegetable peeler.
2. Chop into 1—2 inch chunks.
3. Add to a blender with water. Blend on high for 45—60 seconds.
4. Strain using cheesecloth, a nut milk bag, or fine mesh strainer.
5. Squeeze out all juice and discard pulp.

Sub-Recipe: Homemade Sugarcane Juice (Blender Method)

- 6—8 pieces of sugarcane (4—6 inches each), peeled and chopped
- ½ cup cold water

Instructions

1. Wash and peel all citrus and mint leaves thoroughly
2. Juice lemons and oranges using a juicer of your choice (then strain).
3. Prepare the sugarcane juice using the sub-recipe above
4. In a large pitcher, combine sugarcane juice, lemon juice, orange juice, and water.
5. Stir well, chill if desired, and enjoy fresh!

Pro Tip: Use frozen citrus or coconut water cubes with mint leaves to chill your drink without watering down the glow!

Yield

Approximately 80 ounces (about 10 servings)

Tropical Glow Lemonade continued Storage

- Store in an airtight glass container in the refrigerator.
- Best consumed within **24 to 72 hours** for peak freshness and nutritional value.

Kreatively Kiy's Notes

This is your go-to glow-up juice! With hydrating fresh citrus and mineral-rich sugarcane juice, this lemonade not only quenches your thirst— it supports glowing skin, replenishes electrolytes, and makes a perfect wellness drink any time of day.

Melonberry Zing

Ingredients

- 5 radishes
- 2 cucumbers
- 2 cups strawberries
- 1 pomegranate
- 1 cantaloupe
- 1 papaya

Instructions

1. Wash all produce thoroughly.
2. Peel or core ingredients as needed (e.g., cantaloupe, papaya).
3. Cut larger fruits or vegetables into smaller chunks for easier juicing.
4. Juice all ingredients using a juicer of your choice (then strain).
5. Stir well, chill if desired, and enjoy fresh!

Pro Tip: For a naturally vibrant and slightly spiced kick, slice the radishes and allow them to infuse for 5—10 minutes after juicing.

Serving Size

Approximately 90 ounces (about 9 servings)

Storage

- Store in an airtight glass container in the refrigerator.
- Best consumed within **24 to 72 hours** for peak freshness and nutritional value.

Kreatively Kiy's Notes

Hydrate, glow, repeat *Melonberry Zing* keeps your skin shining as bright as your energy!

Conclusion

As you embark on your juicing journey, remember consistency is key. Start by incorporating one fresh juice into your morning or afternoon routine, prepping ingredients the night before to make it easy and stress-free. Keep your fridge stocked with vibrant fruits and vegetables, and don't be afraid to mix and match flavors to keep things fun and exciting. Set small goals, listen to your body, and let each juice be a reminder that you're choosing wellness - one sip at a time.

Juicing isn't just a trend; it's a lifestyle choice that fuels your body, boosts your energy, and supports long-term health from the inside out. Over time, you'll notice clearer skin, better digestion, improved mood, and a more energized version of yourself ready to take on life creatively and confidently.

At Kreatively Kiy, we believe that when you feel your best, you show up as your best. That's the true power of wellness: it unlocks your potential in every area of life. So, keep pouring into yourself - literally and figuratively - and continue living a Kreatively inspired life, one vibrant juice at a time!

www.ingramcontent.com/pod-product-compliance
Lightning Source LLC
LaVergne TN
LVHW051933051126
851857LV00020B/2085
* 9 7 9 8 9 9 2 3 2 0 4 5 9 *